Hugo Lima de Albuquerque
Antonio Azoubel Antunes
Gabriela Granja Porto

Evaluation of soft tissue thickness in a Brazilian population

Hugo Lima de Albuquerque
Antonio Azoubel Antunes
Gabriela Granja Porto

Evaluation of soft tissue thickness in a Brazilian population

Pilot study

Imprint

Any brand names and product names mentioned in this book are subject to trademark, brand or patent protection and are trademarks or registered trademarks of their respective holders. The use of brand names, product names, common names, trade names, product descriptions etc. even without a particular marking in this work is in no way to be construed to mean that such names may be regarded as unrestricted in respect of trademark and brand protection legislation and could thus be used by anyone.

Cover image: www.ingimage.com

This book is a translation from the original published under ISBN 978-613-9-66709-3.

Publisher:
Sciencia Scripts
is a trademark of
Dodo Books Indian Ocean Ltd. and OmniScriptum S.R.L publishing group

120 High Road, East Finchley, London, N2 9ED, United Kingdom
Str. Armeneasca 28/1, office 1, Chisinau MD-2012, Republic of Moldova, Europe
Printed at: see last page
ISBN: 978-620-8-05810-4

Copyright © Hugo Lima de Albuquerque, Antonio Azoubel Antunes, Gabriela Granja Porto
Copyright © 2024 Dodo Books Indian Ocean Ltd. and OmniScriptum S.R.L publishing group

I dedicate this work to my family, for their support and unconditional love at every moment of my life.

Thank you

I thank God for guiding me this far.

I would like to thank my parents, Euclides Soares de Albuquerque Filho and Maria da Conceição Lima da Silva Albuquerque, for always believing in and supporting my dream. For sacrificing themselves to give me the best education possible. This victory is ours, I love you.

To my brother, Bruno Lima de Albuquerque, for his companionship, support and encouragement. Thank you for helping me at various times, clearing up doubts when I needed it. I love you, Dr Bruno.

To my family dentists, Aunt Márcia Figueirôa, Uncle Marcos Rozendo, for having introduced me to this profession in some way, and to my cousin Jéssica Lahis for her encouragement and support.

To all the teachers and staff at the University of Pernambuco (FOP-UPE) who have contributed in some way to my professional development. Without them, I wouldn't be achieving this goal.

To Prof Dr Gabriela Granja Porto and Prof Dr Antônio Azoubel Antunes, for their guidance during the scientific initiation project and the development of the course completion work. Thank you for your trust and for the knowledge you taught me.

To the radiology department of the Oswaldo Cruz University Hospital (HUOC), for allowing the research to be carried out.

To my friends Huan Soei, José Mário Cassiano and Sebastião Carvalho, for their friendship and support from the beginning to the end of this arduous university journey. You have contributed greatly to my professional and personal growth. You were essential in getting me this far.

To my partner, Gabriel Batista Esteves, who contributed a lot to my learning during the course. Thank you for your patience and friendship.

Many thanks to all of you!

Summary

Purpose: The aim of this study was to compare the thickness of the soft tissues of the face in living people. Material and method: 20 craniometric points in common between the populations compared were selected. The population of Recife- PE/Brazil was compared with other populations, including those from Africa, China, Korea, Slovakia, Colombia and France. The comparison was made using the variables obtained (race, age group, BMI and gender) with those obtained in studies published in the literature. Results: there are differences in the thickness of the soft tissues of the face between the populations studied, with a p-value < 0.05, with the African population standing out in relation to males at the Nasion, Rhinion, Midphiltrum, Supra dental, Pogonion, Mentum, Supra-orbital, Infra-orbital, Lateral orbit, Inferior malar, Zygomatic arch, Supra-glenoid, Supra M2, Occlusal line, Sub M2 points; in females, the points Supra glabella, Nasion, Midphiltrum, Supra dental, Infra dental, Pogonio, Supra orbital, Lateral orbit, Inferior malar, Supra glenoid, Gonio, Supra M2, Occlusal line and Sub M2. With the French population, it was at the points Glabella, Nasion, Supra dental, Infra dental, Supra mental, Mentum, Inferior malar, Zygomatic arch, Supra M2, Sub M2. The Chinese in relation to BMI, the normal men, Supra-glabella, Glabella, Midphiltrum, Infra dental, Supra-orbital, Zygomatic arch, Supra-glenoid, Occlusal line, with overweight was Infra-dental, Pogonio, Lateral orbit and Gonio; female normal BMI had the points Supra dental, Infra dental, Supra mental, Supra glenoid, Supra M2, with overweight the points Supra-glabella and Infra dental. Colombians with a normal BMI had Rhinion, Mento, Supra-orbital, Infra-orbital, Supra-glenoid, and overweight had Mento, Supra-orbital, Infra-orbital, Gonio and Supra M2; women with a normal BMI had Rhinion, Midphiltrum, Mento, Supra-orbital, Supra-glenoid, Supra M2. With the Koreans, the men's points were Nasion, Rhinion, Midphiltrum, Infra dental, Supra-orbital, Supra M2; the women's points were Supra-glabella, Nasion, Rhinion, Midphiltrum, Infra dental, Supra mental, Supra orbital, Supra-glenoid, Gonio, Supra M2, Occlusal line and Sub M2. For Slovaks, males differed in Nasion, Rhinion, Inferior malar, Zygomatic arch, Occlusal line; females in Supra-glabella, Nasion, Rhinion, Inferior malar, Supra-glenoid, Supra M2; for the age group (up to 39 years) of this same population, males differed in Rhinion, Supra-dental and Occlusal line, females in Nasion, Supra dental, Supra M2. Conclusion: Ethnicity influences comparisons of facial soft tissue thickness; there is a difference between the sexes.

Keywords: Race distribution, Age distribution, Computerised tomography, Human identification.

Summary

CHAPTER 1

INTRODUCTION

Nowadays there is a huge demand for individual recognition in both the civil and criminal spheres, as well as for the identification of corpses or skeletons. There are various ways of identifying the individual in each of these situations, depending on whether they are alive or dead in a cadaveric or skeletal stage (FRANCA, 2008).

Thus, more specifically for the identification of human skeletal remains, a variety of methods can be used, such as DNA analysis and radiographs of the teeth (PANENKOVÁ et al., 2012; SIPAHIOGLU; ULUBAY; DIREN, 2012). Although these methods provide important information for forensic scientists regarding the age, sex and body size of the deceased, many of them may not be useful as they depend on the availability of comparative material, either from the police database, dentists or relatives, which can make personal identification impossible (GREEF et aL, 2006; MANHEIN et aL, 2000; PANENKOVÁ et aL, 2012; SIPAHIOGLU; ULUBAY; DIREN, 2012). Facial reconstruction is the last method when other identification methods have failed (SIPAHIOGLU; ULUBAY; DIREN, 2012). The result of this method is an image of the unknown deceased based on the average soft tissue thickness values obtained from specific populations, which can enable an individual to be recognised.

In this way, detailed information obtained from the physiological and osteological analysis of the remains together with data on sex, age and the thickness of the soft tissue in a specific population can promote successful identification.

Data on the thickness of the soft tissue is an integral part of the approaches to obtaining an approximation of the face (STEPHAN, 2006). These paths work on the assumption that the skull morphology is sufficiently distinct and provides an efficient framework for a unique facial appearance even when average soft tissue thickness values are applied.

Recently, the number of studies on this subject has increased. Many methods have been established to measure soft tissue thickness in cadavers and in the living. To this end, many studies have been carried out on cadavers by inserting a calibrated needle into the face at specific points (SUZUKI, 1948; RHINE; CAMPBELL, 1980; SIMPSON; HENNENBERG, 2002; DOMARACKI; STEPHAN, 2006; CODINHA, 2009; TEDESCHI-OLIVEIRA et aL, 2009). Even so, in order to carry out these studies on living people, imaging techniques have been developed that can minimise errors due to changes in *post-mortem* soft tissues when these studies are carried out on cadavers. The imaging methods used in facial thickness studies are: radiography (GARLIE; SAUNDERS, 1999; GEORGE, 1987; SMITH; BUSCHANG, 2001; UTSUNO et al, 2005; UTSUNO et al, 2010), ultrasound (AULSEBROOK; BECKER; ISCAN, 1996; EL-MEHALLAWI; SOLIMAN, 2001; GREEF et al, 2006; LEBEDINSKAYA; VESELOVSKAYA, 1986; MANHEIN et al, 2000; SMITH; THROCKMORTON, 2004; WILKINSON, 2002), magnetic resonance imaging (PLUYM et aL, 2007; SAHNI et aL, 2008; SIPAHIOGLU; ULUBAY; DIREN, 2012) and computerised tomography scans (DONG et aL, 2012; PANENKOVÁ et aL, 2012; PHILIPS; SMUTS, 1996).

Previous studies have shown that different populations exhibit significant variation in soft tissue thickness, and it has been questioned whether data from one population can be applied to the facial reconstruction of another person with different ancestry (DOMARACKI; STEPHAN, 2006; EL-MEHALLAWI; SOLIMAN, 2001; GARLIE; SAUNDERS, 1985; GEORGE, 1987; KASAI, 1998; SIPAHIOGLU; ULUBAY; DIREN, 2012). For this reason, in order to obtain an accurate facial reconstruction, it is necessary to build a database of soft tissue thickness for a specific population. There is available data published in the scientific literature on live facial thickness for the Japanese (SUZUKI, 1948), Portuguese (CODINHA, 2009), Egyptians (EL-MEHALLAWI; SOLIMAN, 2001), Indians (SAHNI et al, 2008), Zulus (AULSEBROOK; BECKER; ISCAN, 1996), mixed populations from South Africa (PHILIPS; SMUTS, 1996), black Americans (RHINE; CAMPBELL, 1980) and Greeks (GREEF et al, 2006). However, it is only found in cadavers in the Brazilian population (TEDESCHI-OLIVEIRA et aL, 2009).

Furthermore, it is not known for sure how different these measurements are and at which craniometric points there is this difference in the various populations around the world. Therefore, this research aimed to compare the database for determining the thickness of the soft tissue of a Brazilian population with the database of other populations around the world in order to see if there is a difference between them or not.

CHAPTER 2

LITERATURE REVIEW

Forensic anthropology is the branch of forensic medicine whose main object is the identity and identification of human beings, and it can also be useful in identifying skeletonised human remains.

Identity is understood to be the set of characteristics that individualise a person, making them distinct from others. It is noteworthy that nowadays the demands for individual recognition, whether in the sphere of civil or criminal life, or in the identification of corpses or skeletons, are enormous. This makes the process of determining a person's identity, known as identification, extremely important in trying to prove that the individual, whether alive or dead, is themselves (FRANÇA, 2008).

2.1 Human identification

2.1.1 General considerations

The history of human identification goes back a long way. The Code of Hammurabi already described a way of identifying criminals: amputation of the ear, nose, fingers or hand, varying according to the degree of the offence. However, over the years and with the consequent humanisation of customs, this type of identification has been replaced by a more scientific one that uses anthropological and anthropometric resources (FRANÇA, 2008).

Identification can be carried out on the living (missing persons, patients with mental disorders, minors, refusal of identity), the dead (mass disasters, unidentified corpses, mutilated corpses, advanced states of putrefaction and cadaveric remains), and the skeleton (decomposition in the skeletonisation phase, skeletons and isolated bones) (FRANÇA, 2008).

This development in the process of *post-mortem* human identification led to the need to organise and standardise the procedures of this process in successive degrees of complexity. This led to the *post-mortem* human identification process being divided into general and individual.

General identification involves the study of various signalling aspects that will form an individual's biotype. These studies begin with the establishment of the animal species, which is carried out through anthropological studies; anatomical comparison of macroscopic aspects with other animals or through anthropometry (FRANÇA, 2008).

Individual identification, on the other hand, is characterised by the need, in most cases, for comparative elements from before the death. For example, in charred bodies, the dental elements are compared with the data in the dental records prior to the events (FRANÇA, 2008).

2.1.2 Human identification on the skeleton

A variety of methods can be used to identify human skeletal remains, such as DNA analysis and radiographs of the teeth (PANENKOVÁ et al., 2012; SIPAHIOGLU; ULUBAY; DIREN, 2012). Although these methods provide important information for forensic scientists regarding the identity of the deceased, many of them may not be useful, because they will depend, in order to be accurate, on the availability of comparative material, either from the police database, dental surgeons or relatives, which may make personal identification impossible (GREEF et al, 2006; MANHEIN et al, 2000; PANENKOVÁ et al, 2012; SIPAHIOGLU; ULUBAY; DIREN, 2012). Facial reconstruction is the last resort when others have not produced the desired identification result (SIPAHIOGLU; ULUBAY; DIREN, 2012).

The aim of forensic facial reconstruction is to recreate, based on the skull, the face of the deceased at the time he/she died, with a sufficient appearance, even if it is not identical, that contributes to its recognition, thus leading to the identification of the body (PANENKOVÁ et aL, 2012). Facial reconstruction does not correspond to a photograph of the individual when alive, but it can be considered a success if it is realistic enough to produce a good response from the public, leading to identification of the individual (TEDESCHI-OLIVEIRA et aL, 2009). The publication of a reconstructed face is expected to encourage family members or friends to recognise the face of a family member who was previously unknown.

2.2 Methods for obtaining facial soft tissue thickness

Facial reconstruction allows the contours of the soft tissues on the skull to be re-established, constructing a face and increasing the likelihood of facial recognition. The reliability of this technique depends on assessing the average values of soft tissue thickness observed in a given population (TEDESCHI-OLIVEIRA et al, 2009).

Identifying the living person or corpse is easier, but not the skeleton. Attempts are made to identify these cases based on characteristics such as age, sex, race, stature and injury marks on the bones. These characteristics can help, but they are not specific enough to indicate that a skull in question belongs to a particular person. Forensic odontology can also establish identity in some cases or provide a possibility in others.

In cases where identifications are difficult, efforts will be made to reconstruct the face from the base of the skull devoid of soft tissue (RHINE; CAMPBELL, 1980; SAHNI et aL, 2008). The fundamental principle for facial reconstructions is to establish the thickness of the soft tissue at a given point on the face and scalp.

In the field of forensic anthropology, all facial reconstruction techniques used in drawings, sculptures and computer-assisted images (MIYASAKA et al., 1995; NELSON; MICHAEL, 1998; UTSUNO et al, 2005; YOSHINO et al, 1997) are based on measuring the thickness of soft tissues so that these measurements can be applied to an as yet unidentified skull in order to obtain a virtual photograph of the individual under investigation (AULSEBROOK; BECKER; ISCAN, 1996; UTSUNO et al, 2005).

Therefore, in order to produce a facial reconstruction, information on the thickness of the soft tissues covering the bony structures of the skull is essential (GARLIE; SAUNDERS, 1999; NELSON; MICHAEL, 1998; TEDESCHI- OLIVEIRA et aL, 2009; TYRRELL et aL, 1997). Vanezis et aL (2000) define soft tissue thickness markers as lines projected from points on the skull to points on the face. The length of these lines corresponds to the thickness of the soft tissue in a particular region.

Bearing in mind that this thickness varies for each ethnic group and that it is questionable whether a specific measurement for one population can be used in another (DOMARACKI; STEPHAN, 2006; EL-MEHALLAWI; GARLIE; SAUNDERS, 1985; KASAI, 1998; SAHNI et al, 2008; SIPAHIOGLU; ULUBAY; DIREN, 2012; SOLIMAN, 2001; SUZUKI, 1948), from the 19th century to the present day, physical anthropologists and forensic scientists have studied various methods that can be used to measure the thickness of soft tissue in cadavers and in the living of numerous distinct populations (AULSEBROOK; BECKER; ISCAN, 1996; DONG et al, 2012; LEBEDINSKAYA; VESELOVSKAYA, 1986; PANENKOVÁ et al, 2012; PHILIPS; SMUTS, 1996; SAHNI et al, 2008; SIPAHIOGLU; ULUBAY; DIREN, 2012; TEDESCHI- OLIVEIRA et al, 2009). These include needle puncture, X-rays, ultrasound, computerised tomography and magnetic resonance imaging

(UTSUNO et aL, 2010).

The first method to be used to check the thickness of the soft tissues of the face in cadavers was the needle. Welcker (1883) was the author accepted as the first to record the depth of soft tissue by inserting a scalpel blade into the tissue at predefined points. This method was slightly modified by His (1895) who used a needle with a piece of rubber on the tip, with the intention that when the needle was pushed into the cadaver's skin, the rubber would be pulled back to represent the depth of the tissue. Kollmann and Buchly (1898) used a needle covered in soot, the "clean" part of the needle representing the depth of the tissue. Susuki (1948) collected facial soft tissue data on Japanese men and Rhine and Campbell (1980) on black American men, both on cadavers using calibrated needles with a rubber bulkhead. However, the needle technique can lead to errors such as inaccurate localisation of points on the surface of the skin, performed by palpation on tissue that has already shrunk after death, which makes it impossible to measure soft tissue thickness correctly (PHILIPS; SMUTS, 1996; UTSUNO et al., 2005).

Other methods used to determine the depth of soft tissue that have allowed live studies to be carried out are radiography, computerised tomography, ultrasound and magnetic resonance imaging (PANENKOVÁ et aL, 2012; SAHNI et aL, 2008). Some researchers have found that all methods have specific errors, and suggest that no method is completely accurate, each of these methods having its own limitations (PANENKOVÁ et aL, 2012; SUZUKI, 1948).

Some studies have used cephalometric radiographs to collect soft tissue data in the living (DUMONT, 1986; GEORGE, 1987), but due to the harmful effects of X-rays, the superimposition of various anatomical structures on the film and not being able to collect bilateral data has made scientists reluctant to use this method for this purpose (AULSEBROOK; BECKER; ISCAN, 1996; LEBEDINSKAYA; VESELOVSKAYA, 1986; MANHEIN et al, 2000; PANENKOVÁ et aL, 2012).

Lebedinskaya and Veselovskaya (1986) began using ultrasound to measure soft tissue depth in Russian adults from various ethnic groups. Hodson, Lieberman and Wright (1985) also studied this method in Caucasoid American children. Although it is a risk-free method because it does not expose the study population to radiation, ultrasound is subject to errors due to variations in the angulation of the ultrasound depth in relation to the bone and the complicated detection of transition points between bone and soft tissue. In addition, when carrying out the examination, pressure is imposed on the soft tissues which can alter the result of the soft tissue thickness (PANENKOVÁ et aL, 2012; PLUYM et aL, 2007).

Phillips and Smuts (1996) used computerised tomography to measure facial soft tissue thickness in a South African population, as did Panenkova et al. (2012) in the Slovak population and Dong et al. (2012) in the Chinese. Despite being a procedure with radiation exposure to individuals, it is precise and makes accurate measurement possible. In order to minimise the harmful effect of radiation on study subjects, many studies have been carried out using examinations with the aim of diagnosing diseases rather than for the specific purpose of the study (PANENKOVÁ et al., 2012).

Magnetic resonance imaging has also been used to measure soft tissue depth in India (SAHNI et al., 2008), Turkey (SIPAHIOGLU; ULUBAY; DIREN, 2012) and Canada (PLUYM et al., 2007). It is favoured by some authors because it has low radiation exposure and satisfactory results, although some errors are inevitable because the image of the bone in this type of examination is dark, which can make it difficult to mark the craniometric points (DONG et aL, 2012).

It is worth noting that soft tissue thickness not only varies according to an individual's ethnic group, but also according to gender and individual nutritional status (DONG et al, 2012; GREEF et al, 2006; RHINE; CAMPBELL, 1980; SAHNI et al, 2008; SUTTON, 1969; SUZUKI, 1948). Many studies have incorporated three types of body categories (slender, normal and obese) with their contributions to soft tissue thickness, and found that body mass index (BMI) was a major contributing factor in determining differences in thickness between individuals (DONG et al., 2012; GREEF et al., 2006; GREEF et al., 2009; RHINE; CAMPBELL, 1980). For this reason, it is recommended that future facial recognition studies should consider BMI to estimate soft tissue thickness (DONG et al, 2012; STARBUCK; WARD, 2007).

2.3 Studies on facial soft tissue thickness

Albuquerque et al (2014) carried out a study in the population of Recife-PE/Brazil and a sample of 30 patients was analysed, of whom 15 were men and 15 were women, of whom 20 (66.7%) called themselves brown, 7 (23.3%) called themselves black and only 3 (10.0%) white. The 20 craniometric points of choice were measured on a computer using the Invesalius 3.0 programme. The variables used in this study were age group, which was divided into patients aged up to 39 and 40 and over, gender, ethnicity, weight, height and

BMI, slender (BMI<20), normal (BMI=20-25) and obese (BMI>25). The results showed that three points had greater soft tissue thickness, primarily Supra M2, the occlusal line and Sub M2. The points with the least thickness were those located on the frontal bone, the Supraglabella, Glabella and Nasion, and the Rhinion in the nose region, with the Rhinion having the least thickness. In relation to gender, the distances or measurements for the pogonion, lateral orbit, zygomatic arch, supra M2 and Sub M2 were higher in females than in males; in the other measurements, the means were correspondingly higher in males; however, there was a significant difference between the sexes ($p < 0.05$) in the distances: Supraglabella, Nasion, Rhinion, Midphiltrum, Supra dental, Infra dental, Lateral orbit and Gonio. For the age group of the Recife population, there was no significant difference. In relation to BMI, the Pogonio measurement was the only one with a significant difference.

For the study of the Chinese population, DONG et al. (2012) used a sample of 200 patients, of whom 75 were men and 125 women of northern Chinese origin, who visited Qindu Hospital and Xijing Hospital. The age of the male subjects ranged from 22 to 29 years, and the age of the female subjects ranged from 18 to 32 years. Gender, height and weight and BMI (containing three ranges, <20, 20-25,> 25) were used as variables. There were 23 males and 42 females in the thin category, 34 males and 64 females in the normal category, and 18 males and 19 females in the obese category. In this study, the greatest soft tissue thickness was identified at reference points located in the cheek region, with the thinnest soft tissue at reference points located on the forehead and in the nasal root region; the maximum was obtained at supra M2, and the minimum was recorded at the rhinion. Overall, the largest measurement ranges were observed in the supra M2 in obese women and normal men, and the smallest measurement ranges were observed in the frontal eminence in the slender category for both sexes. Men showed greater soft tissue thickness measurements than women, except in the glabella, zygomatic arch and supraglenoid in the slender category, supra M2 in the normal category, and gonion, supra M2 and Sub M2 in the obese category. It was shown that only a third of the differences between the sexes were statistically significant.

Perlaza (2013) carried out a study on the Colombian population, the sample also consisted of 30 individuals, 26 (86.7%) males and four (13.3%) females between the ages of 18 and 35. The population included were those of mixed racial origin with descendants in the city of Cali. Seventeen craniometric points were analysed, with weight, height, BMI (underweight, BMI <18.5; normal BMI 18.6-24.9; overweight BMI 25.0-29.9 and obese BMI 30.0) and gender as variables, with p-values < 0.05. In the survey results, no significant differences were found associated with gender for most of the anatomical landmarks; however, where differences were found, these were in the craniometric landmarks in the midline and particularly in the thicker soft tissues in men (the rhinion, supradental, mental eminence, occlusal left line). Supramental was thicker in women. For males with normal nutritional status and overweight, overweight individuals had a significant difference (p <0.05) for the following craniometric points: supradentale, mentum, lower right malar, supra glenoid, Gonio and Sub M2. The Nasion and Rhinion were thicker in normal BMI individuals. Male facial soft tissues were thicker than females for the Rhinion, supra dental, right occlusal line. Female soft tissues were thicker than those of males in the following anatomical structures: rhinion, supradentale, supramental, left infraorbital, right infraorbital, right occlusal line.

In a study of the Slovakian population, Panenková et al, 2012 studied 160 individuals, 80 men and 80 women aged between 18 and 87. The sample was divided into three age groups: 18-39 years, 40-59 years and 60 years. The variables used were the patients' sex and age. Fourteen craniometric points were selected for this study. The median values for facial soft tissue thickness for men exceeded those for women at all 14 reference points, with the exception of the lateral orbit. Statistically significant differences (p <0.05) were observed for nine of the 14 landmarks. Men showed significantly higher soft tissue thickness values in the cheek region (lower malar, occlusal line and supra M2). The landmarks that did not differ significantly between men and women were glabella, rhinion, upper lip margin, infra orbital and zygomatic arch. The comparison between the three age groups of men revealed that soft tissue thickness differed significantly in the supra-glenoid and midphiltum. Thickness in women differed significantly between the three age groups in the glabella, midphiltrum, supraorbital and suborbital.

For the study of the French population, Guyomarc'h et al. (2013) used a sample of 500 patients, obtaining 265 males and 235 females, and an average age of 52 years, between 18 and 96 years. With regard to BMI, this study stated that the average BMI of the French population is 25.3 kg/m2, that obesity tends to be more present in older individuals, and that men are more overweight than women. A BMI of 25 kg / m2 separates the 'normal' group from the overweight group. The proportion of normal (BMI <25) vs. overweight (BMI > 25) individuals is balanced (n = 253 and 247, respectively). The variables gender, age and BMI were used. The study sample shows a significant difference in BMI between men and women. A total of 37 craniometric points were assessed. Age had little effect on tissue thickness and revealed no specific pattern for this variable. The influence of gender was more important and concentrated in the superior and lateral orbital region, the nasal bridge, and the anterosuperior alveolar process. Corpulence tended to strongly influence most soft tissue thicknesses (except for the midline region of the mouth). Almost no interaction effects were detected; according to the authors, this means that the influences of sex, age and BMI are globally independent on soft tissue thickness.

In the Korean population, Hwango et al. (2012) obtained a sample of university students in Gwangju, Korea. All the subjects were of Korean descent, and none of the subjects had undergone orthodontic treatment. Individuals with facial deformities were excluded. Only individuals with a normal BMI were selected. The sample consisted of 100 students, 50 males (age range, 20.2-36.1 years, mean 29.1 years; SD, 3.7 years) and 50 females (age range, 20.0-35.2 years; mean 27.5 years; SD, 4.2 years). Thirty-one craniometric points were compared, 10 in the midline and 21 bilateral points. Only the sex of the individuals studied was used as a variable. When comparing male and female subjects, 18 of the 31 landmarks showed statistically significant differences between the sexes. With regard to gender differences on midline points of interest, six of the 10 locations showed statistically significant differences between male and female subjects. All of them showed higher values in male subjects. In particular, the Midphiltrum, supra dental and infra dental landmarks that correspond to the lip area showed higher values (1.8, 1.8, and 1.4 mm, respectively), indicating a markedly thicker lip in men than in women. In the case of bilateral landmarks, 12 out of 21 sites showed statistically significant differences between the sexes. Although most showed higher values in males, such as the midline landmarks, the lateral orbit corresponding to the zygoma area showed a lower value in males than in females. This indicates that the thickness over the zygoma area is thinner in men than in women, unlike most of the face.

The study in the African population, Philips; Smuts (1996) studied 10 craniometric points in the midline and 11 bilateral points. Thirty-two patients (16 men, 16 women) of mixed racial origin born in the Western Cape province of South Africa were selected for the investigation. Their ages ranged from 12 to 71 years. The study used gender and race as variables and compared them with two other populations. The comparison was made with white and black Americans, and a Japanese population). For this study, only information from the African population was collected, for comparison with the population of Recife/PE (Brazil).

CHAPTER 3

PROPOSAL

17

The aim of the research was to compare a reference database of facial soft tissue thickness in living people from Recife-PE/Brazil with populations from China, Africa, Korea, Slovakia, Colombia and France, according to gender, age group, ethnicity and BMI.

CHAPTER 4

Materials and methods

4.1 Type of study

This research was a comparative study, comparing the thicknesses of the soft tissues of the face in different populations around the world in relation to gender, age, BMI and skin colour.

4.2 Variables

The dependent and independent variables are described in Table 1.

Variable	Descriptor	Category	Aspects
Dependent			
Human identification	Human identification	101.076.368.400 101.198.780.750	Standards
Independent - Thickness of facial soft tissues - Craniometric points - Male - Female - Age	Male Female Distribution by age	101.240.050 N01.224.033 N06.850.505.400.050 SP3.001.037.003	
- Body weight	Body weight	C23.888.144 E01.370.600.115.100.160.120 E05.041.124.160.750 G07.100.100.160.120 G07.700.320.249.314.120 SP6.011.042.048.024	
Distribution by race	Distribution by race	SP3.001.037.023	

Table 1: Description of the dependent and independent variables.

4.3 Sample selection

For the research sample, the pilot study carried out by the authors with a sample of 30 patients was used and the variables obtained (race, age group (up to 39 years and 40 years or more), BMI with slim (BMI<20), normal (BMI=20-25) and obese (BMI> 25) variation and gender) were compared with those obtained in published literature, such as populations in China (DONG et aL, 2012), Africa (PHILIPS; SMUTS, 1996) and the United States (DONG et aL, 2012).25) and gender) with those obtained in studies published in the literature, such as populations in China (DONG et al, 2012), Africa (PHILIPS; SMUTS, 1996), for this study only information was collected from the African population, for comparison with the population of Recife/PE (Brazil), Korea (HWANGO et al, 2012) Slovakia (PANENKOVÁ et al, 2012), Colombia (PERLAZA, 2013) and France (GUYOMARCH et al, 2013).

4.4 Data collection

The studies published in the literature were selected through search engines such as PubMed, Medline, LILACS and SciELO.

Studies were selected to obtain soft tissue thickness in populations that assessed the sex, age, height and weight of the individuals.

We also selected studies that assessed at least 15 of the 20 anthropometric points on the skull (table 1 and figure 1), many of which are standard points used more commonly in the studies found in the literature (DONG et al, 2012; RHINE; CAMPBELL, 1980). Of these, ten are in the midline and ten are bilateral. By anthropometric convention, only the midline points and those on the left side were considered.

Data collection for the population of Recife-PE (ALBUQUERQUE et al, 2014) was carried out at the Oswaldo Cruz University Hospital (HUOC). Patient demand was spontaneous, to avoid unnecessary radiation exposure. The scan was carried out using a 4-channel multislice/GE computerised tomography scanner, with a slice thickness of 1.25mm and an increment of 1mm. This type of scan is capable of producing sectioned, three-plane, 3-dimensional images of an object. The images obtained were viewed in the Invesalius 3.0 software where it was possible to readjust the position and orientation of the head planes and observe the skull and facial surface superimposed.

The measurements were taken perpendicular to the craniometric points according to Vanezis et al. (2000), with the thickness of the soft tissue of the face at a location equal to the length of the projected line from the skeleton to the point of the face in the soft tissue. The measurements will be taken on the monitor using a cursor from the tomography console, with an accuracy of 0.01 mm.

Table 1: Description of the craniometric points considered in this study (DONG et al., 2012).

Mid-sagittal points	Description
1. Supra-glabella	Above the glabella, the most anterior point of the forehead.
2. Glabella	0 most prominent point among the supra-orbital rhymes.
3. *Nasion*	0 midpoint of the suture between the frontal bone and the two nasal bones.
4. *fihinion*	Anterior end of the most anterior point of the nasal bones.
5. *Midphiltrum*	Stitch in the intermaxillary suture, located as far superiorly as possible before the curvature of the beginning of the anterior nasal spine.
6. Supra dental	Between the upper central incisors at the enamel-cement junction.
7. Infra dental	Between the lower central incisors at the enamel-cement junction.
8. Supra mental	Deepest point in the superior sulcus of the mandibular eminence.
9. Pogonio	Most anterior point of the mentonian eminence of the mandible.
10. Mento	Lower point of the mentonian symphysis of the mandible.
Bilateral Points	
11. Supraorbital	Above the orbit, centred on the uppermost edge of the orbit.
12. Infraorbital	Below the orbit, centred on the lower edge of the orbit.
13. Lateral orbit	Alignment of the lateral edge of the eye in the centre of the zygomatic process
14. Lower malar	Centred in the deepest part of the canine fossa.
15. Zygomatic arch	Half the length of the zygomatic arch (most protruded point of the arch when viewed inferosuperiorly).
16. Supra-glenoid	Root of the zygomatic arch, above and anterior to the external auditory meatus.
17. Gonio	Point located on the jaw line at the level of the angle between the posterior and inferior borders of the jaw.
18. Supra M2	Above the upper second molar (if this tooth is lost, the point is placed in the corresponding area).
19. Occlusal line	Point located at the end of the anterior margin of the mandibular ramus in the dental plane of occlusion.
20. Sub M2	Below the lower second molar (if this tooth is lost, the point is placed in the corresponding area).

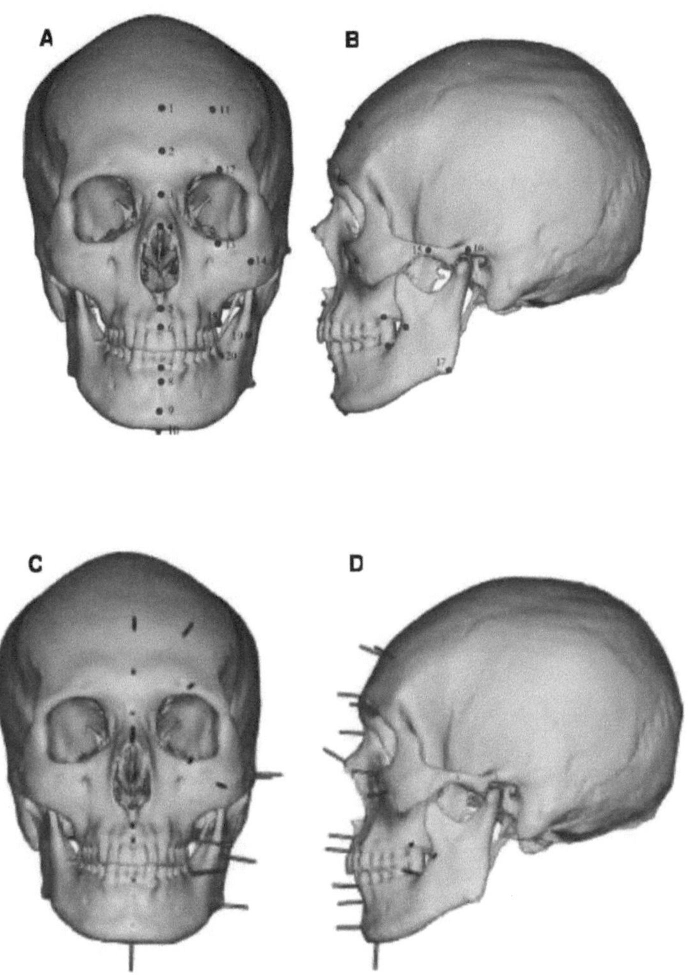

Figure 1 - A and B: Location of craniometric points on frontal and lateral CT scans; C and D: Measurement of thicknesses perpendicular to craniometric points in frontal and lateral views (Source: DONG et aL, 2012).

4.5 Statistical analysis

The paired *i-student* test was used to compare the populations of the mean obtained at each craniometric point.

The significance level used in the statistical test decisions was 5.0% and the programme used to obtain the statistical calculations was SAS *(Statistical Analysis System)* version 8.0 for microcomputers.

4.6 Bioethical considerations

The project was submitted to the ethics committee in order to measure the craniometric points of the 30 patients in the sample. However, another submission to the ethics committee was not necessary in order to make the comparison with other populations.

CHAPTER 5

Results

Table 2 compares the Brazilian population with the Colombian male population with normal BMI. It shows that only 5 of the 17 craniometric points analysed had significant differences. Only 1 point, the chin, had a higher average for the Colombian population. The points that stood out in the Recife population were the Rhinion, Supra-Orbital, Infra-Orbital and Supra-Glenoid. **Table 3**, on the other hand, compares overweight individuals with males. There was also a significant difference between 5 craniometric points, two of which (Mento and Gônio) had a higher average for Colombians, while 3 points prevailed in the Recife population, the Supra-orbital, Infra-orbital and Supra M2.

Table 2 - Comparison between the measurements of the Brazilian and Colombian populations of normal weight males.

Measures	Population Recife Male normal weight		Colombian population Male normal weight		p-value[1]
	Average	DP	Average	DP	
Supra-glabella	5,7	1,3	**	**	**
Glabella	5,5	0,4	**	**	**
Nasion	7,7	1,7	7,1	1,2	0,493
Rhinion	3,6	0,7	2,6	0,4	0,028*
Midphiltrum	15,1	2,6	14,3	2,0	0,518
Supra dental	10,7	2,5	11,7	1,0	0,431
Infra dental	10,3	1,4	11,6	1,0	0,102
Supra mental	13,3	2,2	12,5	1,3	0,486
Pogonio	9,4	1,7	**	**	**
Mento	7,6	1,7	11,7	1,4	0,006*
Supra-orbital	8,4	0,6	6,5	0,9	0,002*
Infraorbital	6,8	1,4	5	0,9	0,042*
Lateral orbit	8,9	1,7	8	1,2	0,298
Lower malar	17,9	2,1	15,8	2,0	0,085
Zygomatic arch	8,3	1,6	8	1,1	0,641
Supra-glenoid	13,4	2,0	10,2	1,0	0,025*
Gonio	13,3	4,4	16,8	2,0	0,154
Supra M2	29,9	5,5	23,6	3,9	0,063
Occlusal line	23,1	2,6	22,9	2,3	0,861
Sub M2	21,3	2,8	21,9	1,9	0,650

(*): Significant difference at 5%.
(**): Missing value in the reference.
(1): Using the one-sample Student's t-test.

Table 3 - Comparison between the measurements of the Brazilian and Colombian male populations among the overweight.

Measures	Population Recife Overweight male		Colombian population Overweight male		p-value[1]
	Average	DP	Average	DP	
Supra-glabella	4,2	1,2	**	**	**
Glabella	6,4	1,3	**	**	**
Nasion	7,0	1,0	6,7	1,2	0,491

Rhinion	4,0	1,4	2,5	0,4	0,073
Midphiltrum	13,3	3,4	14,8	1,4	0,388
Supra dental	12,3	2,2	12,8	2,1	0,662
Infra dental	11,7	1,6	12,5	1,4	0,336
Supra mental	13,1	1,9	11,9	1,1	0,236
Pogonio	13,6	1,7	**	**	**
Mento	10,1	2,2	13,5	1,2	0,025*
Supra-orbital	8,8	2,0	6,2	1,3	0,044*
Infraorbital	8,4	1,4	5,5	1,3	0,010*
Lateral orbit	8,6	0,9	8,6	1,8	0,953
Lower malar	19,5	3,5	17,1	2,2	0,196
Zygomatic arch	7,6	2,3	8,9	2,4	0,262
Supra-glenoid	15,4	3,4	11,9	1,6	0,080
Gonio	12,5	2,9	20,6	4,5	0,003*
Supra M2	33,1	3,2	26,7	3,8	0,011*
Occlusal line	26,0	3,1	23,9	2,1	0,209
Sub M2	23,4	2,5	24,2	2,7	0,523

(*): Significant difference at 5%.
(**): Value missing from the reference.
(1): Using the one-sample Student's t-test.

Table 4 compares females with normal BMI in the Colombian and Brazilian populations. There were 6 craniometric points with a significant difference, 2 of which had a higher mean for Colombian women (Midphiltrum and Mento). The other 4 craniometric points stood out in the Brazilian population (Rhinion, Supra-orbital, Supra-glenoid, Supra M2).

Table 4 - Comparison between the measurements of the Brazilian and Colombian populations of normal weight females.

Measures	Population Recife Female normal weight		Colombian population Female normal weight		p-value[1]
	Average	DP	Average	DP	
Supra-glabella	4,1	0,7	**	**	**
Glabella	6,2	1,1	**	**	**
Nasion	5,8	0,8	6,4	0,4	0,136
Rhinion	2,7	0,6	1,8	0,2	0,026*
Midphiltrum	9,9	0,9	12,9	1,7	0,002*
Supra dental	8,4	1,3	9,7	1,5	0,091
Infra dental	11,3	2,1	10,9	1,4	0,677
Supra mental	13,2	2,9	14,5	1,5	0,368
Pogonio	10,2	2,5	**	**	**
Mento	7,0	2,1	10,7	1,5	0,017*
Supra-orbital	8,1	1,4	5,7	1,1	0,020*
Infraorbital	7,4	1,6	6	0,6	0,126
Lateral orbit	10,3	0,9	9,2	1,5	0,066
Lower malar	17,4	3,3	16,2	1,7	0,461
Zygomatic arch	9,5	4,1	7,9	1,5	0,430
Supra-glenoid	13,3	2,9	9,5	0,6	0,042*
Gonio	18,5	7,0	14,3	2,6	0,250
Supra M2	33,3	3,2	22,4	3,0	0,002*
Occlusal line	23,4	4,9	20,5	0,7	0,266
Sub M2	20,2	7,7	20,7	1,1	0,883

(*): Significant difference at 5%.
(**): Value missing from the reference.
(1): Using the one-sample Student's t-test.

When comparing the Korean male population, **table 5** found 6 (Nasion, Rhinion, Midphiltrum, Infra dental, Supra-orbital, Supra M2) craniometric points with a significant difference. Of the points analysed, only one had a higher average for Koreans, the Infra dental. As for the Korean female population in **Table 6,** of the 20 points assessed, 11 craniometric points showed significant differences (Supra-glabella, Nasion, Rhinion, Midphiltrum, Infra dental, Supra mental, Supra-orbital, Supra-glenoid, Gonio, Supra M2 and Occlusal line). Supra-glabella and Infra-dental had a higher average for Korean women.

Table 5 - Comparison between the measurements of the Brazilian and Korean male populations.

Measures	Population Recife Male		Korean population Male		p-value[1]
	Average	DP	Average	DP	
Supra-glabella	4,7	1,3	5,3	0,7	0,091
Glabella	5,9	1,1	5,6	0,6	0,309
Nasion	7,7	2,0	6,4	0,9	0,020*
Rhinion	3,5	1,0	2,3	0,6	<0,001*
Midphiltrum	14,1	2,7	12,5	1,1	0,039*
Supra dental	11,7	2,2	11,7	2,0	0,973
Infra dental	11,0	1,7	13	1,9	<0,001*
Supra mental	12,4	2,1	11,6	1,1	0,181
Pogonio	10,9	3,1	12.3	1,4	0,101
Mento	8,4	2,5	8.0	1,5	0,543
Supra-orbital	8,4	1,4	7.2	1,1	0,004*
Infraorbital	7,1	1,8	7.4	1,4	0,549
Lateral orbit	8,5	1,5	8.6	1,4	0,775
Lower malar	18,3	2,9	18.6	2,7	0,704
Zygomatic arch	7,9	2,0	8.1	1,7	0,715
Supra-glenoid	13,8	2,9	12.6	2,0	0,126
Gonio	14,3	5,6	14.3	4,0	0,997
Supra M2	31,0	4,1	28.5	2,7	0,035*
Occlusal line	24,1	3,2	22.9	2,6	0,165
Sub M2	22,2	2,5	21.1	2,8	0,106

(*): Significant difference at 5%.
(1): Using the one-sample Student's t-test.

Table 6 - Comparison between the measurements of the Brazilian and Korean female populations.

Measures	Population Recife Female		Korean population Female		p-value[1]
	Average	DP	Average	DP	
Supra-glabella	3,8	0,6	4,8	0,8	<0,001*
Glabella	5,7	1,0	5,3	0,7	0,182
Nasion	6,1	1,2	5,4	0,9	0,034*
Rhinion	2,6	0,7	2,2	0,9	0,040*
Midphiltrum	11,9	2,2	10,7	1,4	0,049*
Supra dental	9,7	2,2	9,9	1,7	0,696
Infra dental	10,3	1,5	11,6	1,6	0,004*
Supra mental	12,2	2,3	10.2	1,1	0,005*
Pogonio	11,2	2,4	12.0	1,8	0,201
Mento	7,6	2,4	6.9	1,5	0,298
Supra-orbital	7,9	1,4	6.4	1,0	0,001*
Infraorbital	6,7	2,3	7.3	1,3	0,338
Lateral orbit	10,6	2,3	10.2	1,4	0,561
Lower malar	17,3	3,2	17.5	2,6	0,830
Zygomatic arch	9,3	2,9	8.7	1,4	0,454
Supra-glenoid	13,1	2,6	11.2	1,8	0,014*
Gonio	19,1	6,5	12.9	2,3	0,002*

Supra M2	33,4	3,5	27.7	3,4	<0,001*
Occlusal line	24,8	4,2	21.2	2,3	0,005*
Sub M2	22,8	5,6	20.3	2,4	0,105

(*): Significant difference at 5%.
(1): Using the one-sample Student's t-test.

As a general comparison of the male sex of the Slovak and Brazilian populations, **table 7** shows five craniometric points with significant differences. The Rhinion and lower malar prevailed for the Recife population, while the Nasion, zygomatic arch and occlusal line had a higher average for the Slovaks. For the female population, as shown in **table 8,** 6 points were seen with a significant difference. The Supra-glabella and Nasion had a higher mean for women from Slovakia. The Rhinion, Inferior Malar, Supra-glenoid and Supra M2 had a higher mean for the Recife population.

Table 7 - Comparison between the measurements of the Brazilian and Slovak male populations.

Measures	Population Recife Male		Slovak population Male		p-value[1]
	Average	DP	Average	DP	
Supra-glabella	4,7	1,3	5,1	1,2	0,246
Glabella	5,9	1,1	5,9	1,3	1,000
Nasion	7,7	2,0	8	1,5	0,003*
Rhinion	3,5	1,0	2,5	0,7	0,002*
Midphiltrum	14,1	2,7	15,2	2,6	0,120
Supra dental	11,7	2,2	12,9	1,9	0,055
Infra dental	11,0	1,7	**	**	**
Supra mental	12,4	2,1	**	**	**
Pogonio	10,9	3,1	**	**	**
Mento	8,4	2,5	**	**	**
Supra-orbital	8,4	1,4	8,2	1,6	0,548
Infraorbital	7,1	1,8	7	2,1	0,812
Lateral orbit	8,5	1,5	9	2,0	0,209
Lower malar	18,3	2,9	16,4	2,5	0,025*
Zygomatic arch	7,9	2,0	9,5	2,4	0,009*
Supra-glenoid	13,8	2,9	13,6	2,6	0,761
Gonio	14,3	5,6	**	**	**
Supra M2	31,0	4,1	30,6	5,2	0,738
Occlusal line	24,1	3,2	26,8	3,7	0,005*
Sub M2	22,2	2,5	**	**	**

(*): Significant difference at 5%.
(**): Missing value in the reference.
(1): Using the one-sample Student's t-test.

Table 8 - Comparison between the measurements of the Brazilian and Slovak female populations.

Measures	Population Recife Female		Slovak population Female		p-value[1]
	Average	DP	Average	DP	
Supra-glabella	3,8	0,6	4,6	0,9	<0,001*
Glabella	5,7	1,0	5,5	1,0	0,537
Nasion	6,1	1,2	6,9	1,2	0,018*
Rhinion	2,6	0,7	2,1	0,6	0,013*
Midphiltrum	11,9	2,2	12,4	2,0	0,402
Supra dental	9,7	2,2	11,4	1,9	0,008
Infra dental	10,3	1,5	**	**	**
Supra mental	12,2	2,3	**	**	**
Pogonio	11,2	2,4	**	**	**
Mento	7,6	2,4	**	**	**
Supra-orbital	7,9	1,4	7,2	1,3	0,072

Measures	Average	DP	Average	DP	p-value
Infraorbital	6,7	2,3	6,8	2,5	0,899
Lateral orbit	10,6	2,3	10	2,0	0,363
Lower malar	17,3	3,2	15,2	2,5	0,021*
Zygomatic arch	9,3	2,9	9,1	2,5	0,818
Supra-glenoid	13,1	2,6	11,5	2,0	0,033*
Gonio	19,1	6,5	**	**	**
Supra M2	33,4	3,5	28,1	4,8	<0,001*
Occlusal line	24,8	4,2	22,6	3,3	0,059
Sub M2	22,8	5,6	**	**	**

(*): Significant difference at 5%.
(**): Value missing from the reference.
(1): Using the one-sample Student's t-test.

Table 9 also shows males aged up to 39 compared to the population of Slovakia. Only three craniometric points differed significantly. The Rhinion was higher for the Recife population and the Supra dental and Occlusal Line had a higher mean for the Slovaks. For females, **table 10** also shows three points with significant differences: the Nasion and the Supra dental for the Slovaks and only the Supra M2 stood out for the Recife population.

Table 9 - Comparison between the measurements of the Brazilian and Slovak populations in males aged up to 39 years.

Measures	Population Recife Male up to 39 years old		Slovak population Male up to 39 years old	p-value[1]
	Average	DP	Average	
Supra-glabella	4,8	1,4	4.6	0,731
Glabella	5,4	0,7	5.3	0,555
Nasion	7,7	1,3	7.5	0,738
Rhinion	3,1	0,7	2.1	0,004*
Midphiltrum	14,7	2,3	15.1	0,651
Supra dental	12,3	2,0	14.0	0,033*
Infra dental	11,0	2,1	**	**
Supra mental	12,6	2,6	**	**
Pogonio	9,8	3,0	**	**
Mento	7,9	2,8	**	**
Supra-orbital	8,5	1,6	7.8	0,208
Infraorbital	6,5	1,8	6.7	0,718
Lateral orbit	8,5	1,8	8.4	0,821
Lower malar	18,6	2,7	15.5	0,009
Zygomatic arch	8,0	2,0	9.3	0,094
Supra-glenoid	12,9	2,3	12.9	0,959
Gonio	13,5	2,8	**	**
Supra M2	31,1	4,9	31.1	0,999
Occlusal line	23,8	3,6	26.7	0,024*
Sub M2	22,5	2,3	**	**

(*): Significant difference at 5%.
(**): Missing value in the reference.
(1): Using the one-sample Student's t-test.

Table 10 - Comparison between the measurements of the Brazilian and Slovak populations in females aged up to 39 years.

Measures	Population Recife Female up to 39 years old		Slovak population Female up to 39 years old	p-value[1]
	Average	DP	Average	
Supra-glabella	4,0	0,9	4.3	0,429
Glabella	5,8	1,4	5.0	0,257
Nasion	5,4	0,9	6.8	0,027*
Rhinion	2,1	0,7	2.0	0,682
Midphiltrum	11,5	2,0	13.4	0,109

Measures	Average	DP	Average	p-value
Supra dental	9,1	1,4	11.8	0,011*
Infra dental	9,6	1,0	**	**
Supra mental	11,7	1,9	**	**
Pogonio	10,1	2,0	**	**
Mento	7,4	2,3	**	**
Supra-orbital	7,5	1,3	6.7	0,262
Infraorbital	6,2	2,2	5.2	0,361
Lateral orbit	9,4	1,6	9.4	0,987
Lower malar	18,1	3,1	14.6	0,061
Zygomatic arch	9,8	4,1	7.9	0,359
Supra-glenoid	12,3	3,5	10.8	0,398
Gonio	20,3	6,9	**	**
Supra M2	31,5	3,8	26.6	0,045*
Occlusal line	25,9	3,9	21.5	0,065
Sub M2	25,5	3,9	**	**

(*): Significant difference at 5%.
(**): Value missing from the reference.
(1): Using the one-sample Student's t-test.

Table 11 shows the comparison with the African male population. Of the 20 points analysed, only 1 point had a higher average in Africans (Supra dental). The other 14 points (Nasion, Rhinion, Midphiltrum, Pogonio, Mento, Supra-orbital, Infra-orbital, Lateral orbit, Inferior malar, Zygomatic arch, Supra-glenoid, Supra M2, Occlusal line, Sub M2) had higher averages for the Recife population. For females, in **Table 12,** 14 points had significant differences. Of these points, 3 had higher averages in Africans (Supra-glabella, Supra-dental and Infra-dental); the other 11 craniometric points stood out for the Recife population.

Table 11 - Comparison between the measurements of the Brazilian population and the African population in males.

Measures	Population Recife Male		African population Male		p-value[1]
	Average	DP	Average	DP	
Supra-glabella	4,70	1,28	5.36	1,44	0,066
Glabella	5,90	1,09	5.47	0,68	0,149
Nasion	7,73	1,96	4.00	2,42	<0,001*
Rhinion	3,52	1,04	2.88	1,08	0,032*
Midphiltrum	14,06	2,66	12.25	2,97	0,020*
Supra dental	11,72	2,19	13.16	2,51	0,023*
Infra dental	11,04	1,67	10.43	1,69	0,182
Supra mental	12,35	2,07	12.02	2,07	0,545
Pogonio	10,92	3,05	8.94	2,42	0,025*
Mento	8,41	2,53	6.61	1,71	0,016*
Supra-orbital	8,42	1,38	5.46	1,31	<0,001*
Infraorbital	7,11	1,81	5.97	2,87	0,028*
Lateral orbit	8,49	1,51	7.54	1,49	0,030*
Lower malar	18,31	2,94	0.00	0,00	<0,001*
Zygomatic arch	7,90	2,03	6.49	2,50	0,017*
Supra-glenoid	13,84	2,94	9.10	4,04	<0,001*
Gonio	14,30	5,63	14.20	6,08	0,949
Supra M2	30,96	4,08	12.68	2,10	<0,001*
Occlusal line	24,09	3,15	19.06	9,08	<0,001*
Sub M2	22,21	2,49	13.13	5,31	<0,001*

(*): Significant difference at 5%.
(1): Using the one-sample Student's t-test.

Table 12 - Comparison between the measurements of the Brazilian population and the African population in females.

Measures	Population Recife Female		African population Female		p-value[1]
	Average	DP	Average	DP	
Supra-glabella	3,83	0,61	4.88	1,02	<0,001*
Glabella	5,66	1,01	5.64	1,42	0,926
Nasion	6,10	1,15	4.68	2,35	<0,001*
Rhinion	2,59	0,67	2.78	0,91	0,290
Midphiltrum	11,91	2,18	10.13	2,48	0,007*
Supra dental	9,68	2,15	13.63	3,70	<0,001*
Infra dental	10,27	1,50	12.45	2,31	<0,001*
Supra mental	12,18	2,34	11.70	1,66	0,438
Pogonio	11,17	2,39	9.57	2,36	0,021*
Mento	7,57	2,41	6.47	1,57	0,098
Supra-orbital	7,90	1,39	5.79	1,89	<0,001*
Infraorbital	6,73	2,25	6.42	3,83	0,607
Lateral orbit	10,55	2,25	8.25	2,52	0,001*
Lower malar	17,32	3,15	0.00	0,00	<0,001*
Zygomatic arch	9,28	2,89	9.30	3,21	0,974
Supra-glenoid	13,06	2,55	8.44	3,84	<0,001*
Gonio	19,11	6,47	13.50	6,60	0,005*
Supra M2	33,38	3,50	12.99	4,45	<0,001*
Occlusal line	24,82	4,18	21.26	8,37	0,005*
Sub M2	22,82	5,64	11.88	5,95	<0,001*

(*): Significant difference at 5%.
(1): Using the one-sample Student's t-test.

Table 13 shows a generalised comparison of the thicknesses of the points between the Recife and French populations. Of the 14 craniometric points analysed, 8 (Glabella, Nasion, Supra dental, Infra dental, Mento, Zygomatic Arch, Supra M2 and Sub M2) obtained a higher average for the French population and only 2 (Supra mental and Malar inferior) for the Recife population, with 10 points showing a significant difference.

Table 13- Comparison between the measurements of the Brazilian and French populations in terms of general data.

Measures	Population Recife		French population		p-value[1]
	Average	DP	Average	DP	
			**	**	**
Supra-glabella	4,3	1,1			
Glabella	5,8	1,0	6.5	1,2	0,001*
Nasion	6,9	1,8	8.2	1,6	<0,001*
Rhinion	3,1	1,0	3.0	0,9	0,757
Midphiltrum	13,0	2,6	12.9	2,8	0,857
Supra dental	10,7	2,4	14.1	2,5	<0,001*
Infra dental	10,7	1,6	16.8	3,1	<0,001*
Supra mental	12,3	2,2	9.4	2,1	<0,001*
Pogonio	11,0	2,7	11.8	2,1	0,135
Mento	8,0	2,5	9.5	3,3	0,002*
Supra-orbital	8,2	1,4	**	**	**
Infraorbital	6,9	2,0	**	**	**
Lateral orbit	9,5	2,2	**	**	**
Lower malar	17,8	3,0	14.9	3,2	<0,001*
Zygomatic arch	8,6	2,6	10.0	2,1	0,005*
Supra-glenoid	13,5	2,7	**	**	**
Gonio	16,7	6,4	18.5	6,9	0,137
Supra M2	32,2	3,9	34.5	5,0	0,003*

Occlusal line	24,5	3,7	**	**	**
Sub M2	22,5	4,3	27.7	5,3	<0,001*

(*): Significant difference at 5%.
(**): Missing value in the reference.
(1): Using the one-sample Student's t-test.

When comparing the Chinese population with the Brazilian population, **table 14** shows males with normal BMI. It was seen that of the 9 points with a significant difference, only 1 point (Infra dental) had a higher average for the Chinese, the other 8 (Supra-glabella, Glabella, Rhinion, Midphiltrum, Supra-orbital, Zygomatic arch, Supra-glenoid, Occlusal line) craniometric points had a higher average for the Recife population. As for the overweight male population, in **Table 15,** only 4 points had a significant difference. The Infra dental, Lateral Orbit and Gonion points had higher means for individuals of Yellow ethnicity and only the Pogonion had a higher mean for the Recife population.

Table 14 - Comparison between the measurements of the Brazilian and Chinese populations for males with normal nutritional status.

Measures	Population Recife Male normal weight		Chinese Population Male normal weight		p-value[1]
	Average	DP	Average	DP	
Supra-glabella	5,67	1,28	4.01	0,73	0,045*
Glabella	5,50	0,38	4.59	0,76	0,006*
Nasion	7,68	1,72	5.98	1,25	0,092
Rhinion	3,58	0,65	2.58	0,54	0,026*
Midphiltrum	15,12	2,59	11.64	2,33	0,040*
Supra dental	10,72	2,50	12.68	2.02	0,155
Infra dental	10,28	1,39	14.57	2,26	0,002*
Supra mental	13,26	2,22	10.63	1,24	0,057
Pogonio	9,40	1,65	10.32	2,24	0,281
Mento	7,58	1,71	6.99	1,45	0,483
Supra-orbital	8,43	0,57	6.76	1,37	0,003*
Infraorbital	6,80	1,37	7.18	2,12	0,570
Lateral orbit	8,90	1,67	10.34	2,35	0,084
Lower malar	17,91	2,07	**	**	**
Zygomatic arch	8,35	1,55	5.48	1,16	0,014*
Supra-glenoid	13,37	2,01	10.79	1,89	0,046*
Gonio	13,33	4,43	13.50	3,02	0,935
Supra M2	29,88	5,49	25.35	4,29	0,139
Occlusal line	23,12	2,59	18.93	3,24	0,022*
Sub M2	21,28	2,83	19.69	3,45	0,277

(*): Significant difference at 5%.
(**): Missing value in the reference.
(1): Using the one-sample Student's t-test.

Table 15 - Comparison between the measurements of the Brazilian and Chinese populations for overweight males (BMI > 25 to 29.99).

Measures	Population Recife Overweight male		Chinese population Overweight male		p-value[1]
	Average	DP	Average	DP	
Supra-glabella	4,22	1,24	4.85	1,12	0,319
Glabella	6,45	1,31	5.68	1,27	0,262
Nasion	7,03	,96	6.77	1,18	0,584
Rhinion	3,98	1,36	3.34	0,88	0,355
Midphiltrum	13,34	3,38	12.66	2,32	0,678
Supra dental	12,35	2,16	14.57	2,25	0,083
Infra dental	11,74	1,56	16.69	2,68	0,002*

Measures	Average	DP	Average	DP	p-value
Supra mental	13,10	1,93	11.31	1,94	0,107
Pogonio	13,59	1,75	10.82	2,36	0,024*
Mento	10,07	2,19	8.98	2,05	0,330
Supra-orbital	8,75	1,96	7.82	1,69	0,350
Infraorbital	8,39	1,40	8.30	2,31	0,889
Lateral orbit	8,57	,93	12.32	2,35	0,001*
Lower malar	19,51	3,48	**	**	**
Zygomatic arch	7,58	2,27	7.97	1,39	0,718
Supra-glenoid	15,41	3,37	11.78	2,82	0,073
Gonio	12,49	2,92	16.69	3,18	0,032*
Supra M2	33,07	3,18	29.54	4,87	0,068
Occlusal line	25,98	3,12	22.98	3,65	0,097
Sub M2	23,41	2,53	23.67	4,21	0,830

(*): Significant difference at 5%.
(**): Missing value in the reference.
(1): Using the one-sample Student's t-test.

Table 16 shows the comparison between the Recife and Chinese female population with normal BMI. It can be seen that only 5 of the points analysed had a significant difference. The Chinese population had a higher average for Supra dental and Infra dental. The Recife population stood out for the Supra mental, Supra glenoid and Supra M2 points.

Table 17 compares overweight females. The analysis showed that only the Supraglabella and Infra dental points showed significant differences, with the average of the two points being higher for the Chinese population.

Table 16 - Comparison between the measurements of the Brazilian and Chinese populations for females with normal nutritional status.

Measures	Population Recife Normal weight female		Chinese population Normal weight females		p-value[1]
	Average	DP	Average	DP	
Supra-glabella	4,09	0,72	3.82	0,81	0,446
Glabella	6,23	1,09	4.55	0,71	0,026
Nasion	5,76	0,77	5.61	1,32	0,685
Rhinion	2,67	0,57	2.47	0,59	0,474
Midphiltrum	9,88	0,92	9.97	1,65	0,828
Supra dental	8,42	1,30	11.55	1,93	0,006*
Infra dental	11,31	2,07	14.37	2,14	0,030*
Supra mental	13,18	2,91	9.39	1,46	0,044*
Pogonio	10,16	2,46	9.29	2,15	0,474
Mento	6,99	2,12	6.37	0,98	0,548
Supra-orbital	8,11	1,44	6.42	1,09	0,059
Infraorbital	7,40	1,62	6.25	1,35	0,188
Lateral orbit	10,25	0,93	9.65	1,74	0,224
Lower malar	17,40	3,30	**	**	**
Zygomatic arch	9,51	4,09	5.41	1,08	0,089
Supra-glenoid	13,34	2,91	9.69	1,67	0,049*
Gonio	18,50	6,99	12.97	2,85	0,151
Supra M2	33,29	3,21	26.76	3,79	0,010*
Occlusal line	23,35	4,94	17.23	3,17	0,050
Sub M2	20,16	7,72	19.32	3,14	0,820

(*): Significant difference at 5%.
(**): Value missing from the reference.
(1): Using the one-sample Student's t-test.

Table 17 - Comparison between the measurements of the Brazilian and Chinese populations for overweight females (BMI > 25 to 29.99).

Measures	Population Recife Overweight female		Chinese Population Overweight Females		p-value[1]

	Average	DP	Average	DP	
Supra-glabella	3,54	0,56	4.68	1,14	0,004*
Glabella	5,08	1,05	5.65	0,87	0,238
Nasion	6,54	1,49	6.42	1,27	0,848
Rhinion	2,67	0,88	3.02	0,74	0,370
Midphiltrum	13,16	2,30	11.24	1,94	0,096
Supra dental	10,71	2,42	12.87	2,16	0,081
Infra dental	9,58	0,92	15.58	2,23	<0,001*
Supra mental	11,35	1,93	10.87	1,98	0,567
Pogonio	11,84	2,99	10.61	2,34	0,362
Mento	8,10	2,98	8.59	1,67	0,706
Supra-orbital	7,20	1,16	7.29	1,68	0,861
Infraorbital	5,95	2,82	7.91	1,77	0,149
Lateral orbit	10,64	3,10	11.68	2,17	0,448
Lower malar	17,06	4,06	**	**	**
Zygomatic arch	8,68	2,84	7.88	1,21	0,522
Supra-glenoid	12,90	3,23	10.34	1,95	0,110
Gonio	18,90	6,85	17.21	3,26	0,573
Supra M2	32,12	3,82	30.13	4,58	0,259
Occlusal line	23,82	3,83	22.64	4,15	0,485
Sub M2	22,75	4,66	24.04	3,98	0,529

(*): Significant difference at 5%.
(**): Value missing from the reference.
(1): Using the one-sample Student's t-test.

CHAPTER 6

Discussion

It is remarkable that nowadays the demands for individual recognition, whether in civil or criminal life, or in the identification of corpses or skeletons, are enormous. This makes the process of determining a person's identity, known as identification, extremely important in trying to prove that the individual, whether alive or dead, is themselves (FRANÇA, 2008).

As mentioned in the literature review, there are various methods for obtaining the thickness of the soft tissues of the face. These methods arose from the need to identify individuals, whether living or dead. Initially, the needle puncture technique was used on cadavers, but it was realised that there were changes in soft tissue thickness due to post-mortem dehydration. With the advance of technology, computerised tomography, magnetic resonance imaging, ultrasound and radiography equipment were developed.

The images obtained for use in the research were from CT scans, as they allow the visualisation of bone and soft tissue structures, enabling 3D (three-dimensional) reconstruction of the patient's skull to be carried out using the tomographic slices, thus providing an approximation of the characteristics of the individual's face, with the advantage of being able to take measurements of soft tissue thickness whenever necessary.

This comparative study compared the population of Recife - PE (Brazil) with the populations of Colombia, Korea, Slovakia, Africa, France and China. Both populations were measured using computerised tomography. A difficulty in this regard was the sample size of the Recife-PE population, which was 30 patients (ALBUQUERQUE et al., 2014). The Colombian population also had a sample of 30 patients (PERLAZA, 2013), the French had a sample of 500 patients (GUYOMARC'H et al., 2013), 100 patients were involved in the Korean population (HWANGO et al., 2012), there were 200 patients in China (DONG et al., 2012), the Africans had a sample of 32 patients (PHILIPS; SMUTS, 1996) and the Slovakian population had a sample of 160 individuals (PANENKOVÁ et al., 2012).

During the analysis of the results, it was found that the population of Recife had differences in relation to soft tissue thickness compared to white individuals, the French population (GUYOMARCH et al., 2013) and Slovakia (PANENKOVÁ et al., 2012), black

Africans (PHILIPS; SMUTS, 1996), and yellow Chinese (DONG et al., 2013), 2013) and Slovakia (PANENKOVÁ et al., 2012), black Africans (PHILIPS; SMUTS, 1996), yellow Chinese (DONG et al., 2012) and Koreans (HWANGO et al., 2012), as well as the population of Colombia (PERLAZA, 2013). Black Africans had the greatest significant difference with 15 different craiometric points.

When comparing the populations in terms of body mass index (BMI) and age group, there were no major differences in the thickness of the soft tissues of the face. The items that stood out most were gender and skin colour (race) between the populations compared.

When analysing the Brazilian population with the Colombian population (PERLAZA, 2013), it was found that for men with a normal BMI, the thickness of the soft tissue was greater in 3 bilateral craniometric points, while the Colombian men only had a larger chin compared to the Recife population. In relation to the overweight individuals in these two populations, of the median sagittal points, only the chin had a greater difference, being greater for the Colombians. The Supra-orbital and Infra-orbital points stood out in the Recife population (ALBUQUERQUE et al., 2014), with a higher average (tables 2 and 3). The chin stood out for Colombian men. For normal BMI females (table 4), the chin also stood out for the Colombian population, while the Recife women stood out in 3 bilateral craniometric points, the Supra-orbital, Supra-glenoid and Supra M2 and the median sagittal Rhinion point was higher for the Brazilian women. When comparing these two populations, it was realised that a more prominent chin is a characteristic of Colombians. The Brazilian population claims to be miscegenated, but it is understandable that, due to the historical process of the formation of Brazilian society, the country's population is characterised by a rich ethnic and racial diversity. However, this is a difficulty in this research, as the criterion of racial self-determination adopted by the IBGE makes it difficult to accurately discern the ethnic origins of the population (INSTITUTO BRASILEIRO DE GEOGRAFIA E ESTATÍSICA, 2006). As a result, it is not possible to specify or state with certainty the real ethnicity (miscegenation) of the population.

With regard to the difference in the lower third of the face between Brazilians and Colombians in relation to the chin, a craniometric point that stood out in the Colombian population, an explanation for this finding can be found in a study by Santana et al. (2009). The authors state that the Brazilian group has a more convex profile, with less protrusion of the malar bone, less exposure of the upper incisors and a less protruded chin; the mentolabial sulcus is less pronounced and the soft tissues of the chin are less protruded.

Brazilians form one of the most heterogeneous populations in the world, the result of five centuries of intense miscegenation between peoples from three continents, European colonisers, mainly Portuguese, African slaves and Amerindians who already inhabited these lands. In studies carried out by analysing the mitochondrial DNA of individuals in the four main regions of Brazil, a predominance of Amerindians was observed in the Amazon Region, African lineages in the Northeast, the Southeast in balance, and a European dominance in the South, but the colour of a person's skin alone is not enough to reveal how mixed the population is (PARRA et al., 2003). Even so, the population of north-eastern Brazil, although with a predominance of African lineages, had 15 craniometric points in men and 14 in women that differed from Africans, which was not to be expected. This finding indicates a need to carry out studies with a larger sample in this region in order to accurately assess the predominant lineages of the NE.

In a study of the Korean population (HWANGO et aL, 2012), there was a huge difference for females, with 11 craniometric points having a higher average for Brazilian women, and only two of the points that stood out, the supra-glabella and the infra-dental, were higher for Korean women. For men, the difference was smaller, with only 6 significantly different points, the infra-dental being the only point that stood out for Korean men. It can therefore be seen that when comparing a yellow ethnic population with a mixed race Brazilian population, there are differences, which is considerable for human identification (tables 5 and 6).

For the population of Slovakia (PANENKOVÁ et aL, 2012), the comparison for sex showed significant differences for men in 5 craniometric points, the nasion, zogomatic arch and occlusal line (higher for men from Slovakia), the Rhinion and the lower malar (higher for men from Recife). For females, 6 points had significant differences, most of which were greater for women in Recife. No significant differences were found when comparing age groups.

When compared to the African population (PHILIPS; SMUTS, 1996), the population of Recife (ALBUQUERQUE, H.L., 2014) obtained higher averages. When comparing the Brazilian population with the African population, where black ethnicity prevails, 15 craniometric points had results with significant differences when comparing soft tissue thickness. For males, only the Supra dental point obtained a higher mean with a significant value for Africans. For females, 14 points were significantly different, with only 3 points having higher averages for the African population, the Supra-glabella, the Supra-dental and the Infra-dental, while the other points were higher for the Recife population.

For the French population (GUYOMARCH et aL, 2013), the populations were compared in general and it was observed that 10 craniometric points were significantly different. The French population stood out with a higher average in 8 measurements, only the Supra mental and the Malar inferior were higher for the Brazilian population.

In order to compare the Brazilian and Chinese populations (DONG et aL, 2012), tables were drawn up focussing on the nutritional status of the individuals. Evaluating male individuals with normal BMI, it was observed that there was a significant difference in 9 points of those surveyed, only 1 point was higher for the Chinese, the Infra-dentaL In relation to females with normal BMI, only 5 relevant points were obtained, with the supra dental and infra dental being higher in the Chinese, while the Supra mental, Supra-glenoid and Supra M2 were higher for the Recife population. For overweight men, there was little difference, only 4 points were highlighted out of the 20 points analysed. And for overweight females, only 2 points were significant, which probably doesn't allow us to differentiate between these individuals when considering the BMI variable. This finding is not in line with Starbuck and Ward (2007) who analysed the effects of variations in tissue depths in facial reconstruction through the nutritional status of the individuals, who were thin, normal and obese. BMI influences the thickness of soft tissue in a given population.

The findings of this study show that ethnicity influenced comparisons of facial soft tissue thickness. For this reason, it is necessary to extend this study of soft tissue thickness evaluation to other populations, as it is important for identifying individuals.

CHAPTER 7

Conclusion

With this work, it was possible to see the difference between ethnicities. A comparison was made between individuals of white, black and yellow ethnicity. It was concluded that:

a) **Ethnicities influence comparisons of facial soft tissue thickness;**
b) **There is a difference between the sexes in the different populations.**

BIBLIOGRAPHICAL REFERENCES

ALBUQUERQUE, H.L.; PORTO, G.G.; Scientific initiation research, 2014.

AULSEBROOK, W. A.; BECKER, P. J.; ISCAN, M. Y. Facial softtissue thickness in the adult male Zulu. **Forensic Sei Int,** Ireland, v.79, p.83-102, 1996.

CODINHA, S. Facial soft tissue thicknesses for the Portuguese adult population. **Forensic Sei Int,** Ireland, v.184, p.80.e1-80.e7, 2009.

DOMARACKI, M.; STEPHAN, C. N. Facial soft tissue thickness in Australian adult cadavers. **J Forensic Sei,** Massachusetts, v.51, p.5-10, 2006.

DONG, Y.; HUANG, L.; FENG, Z.; BAI, S.; WUA, G.; ZHAO, Y. Influence of sex and body mass Index on facial soft tissue thickness measurements of the northern Chinese adult population. **Forensic Sei Int,** Ireland, v.222, p.396.e1-396.e7, 2012.

DUMONT, E. R. Mid facial tissue depths of white children: an aid in facial feature reconstruction. **J Forensic Sei,** Massachusetts, v.31, p.1463-1469,1986.

EL-MEHALLAWI, I. H.; SOLIMAN, E. M. Ultrasonicassessmentof facial softtissue thicknesses in adult Egyptians. **Forensic Sei Int,** Ireland, v.117, p.99-107, 2001.

FRANÇA, G. V. **Medicina Legal**. 8ª ed, Rio de Janeiro: Guanabara Koogan, 2008.

GARLIE, T. N.; SAUNDERS, S. R. Midline facial tissue thickness of subadults from longitudinal radiographic study. **J Forensic Sei,** Massachusetts, v.30, p.1100-1112, 1985.

GARLIE, T. N.; SAUNDERS, S. R. Midline facial tissue thicknesses of subadults from longitudinal radiographic study. **J Forensic Sei,** Massachusetts, v.44, p.61-67, 1999.

GEORGE, R. M. The lateral craniographic method of facial reconstruction. **J Forensic Sei,** Massachusetts, v.35, p.1305-1330, 1987.

GREEF, S.; CLAES, P.; VANDERMEULEN, D.; MOLLEMANS, W.; SUETENS, P.; WILLEMS, G. Large-scale in-vivo Caucasian facial soft tissue thickness database for craniofacial reconstruction. **Forensic Sei Int,** Ireland, V.159S1, p.S126-S146, 2006.

GREEF, S.; VANDERMEULEN, D.; CLAES, P.; SUETENS, P.; WILLEMS, G. The influence of sex, age and body mass index on facial soft tissue depths. **Forensic Sei Med Pathol,** New Jersey, v.5, p.60-65, 2009.

GUYOMARCH, P.; SANTOS, F.; DUTAILLY, B.; COQUEUGNIOT, H. Facial soft tissue depths in French adults: Variability, specificity and estimation. **Forensic Sei Int,** Ireland v. 231, p. 411.e1-411.e10,2013.

HIS, W. Anatomische Forschungen ueber Johann Sebastien Bach's gebeine und antlitz nebst Bemerkungen ueber dessen bolder, Abhandlungen der Mathematisch-Physikalischen Klasse der konigl. Sachsischen Gesellschafi der Wissenschafien, v.22, p.379-420, 1895. In: SAHNI, D.; SANJEEV; SINGH, G.; JIT, I.; SINGH, P. Facial soft tissue thickness in northwest Indian adults. **Forensic Sei Int,** v.176, p.137-146, 2008.

HODSON, G.; LIEBERMAN, L. S.; WRIGHT, P. In vivo measurements of facial tissue thicknesses in American Caucasoid children. **J Forensic Sei,** Massachusetts, v.30, p.1100-1112, 1985.

HWANG, H.; PARK, M.; LEE, W.; CHO, J.; KIM, B.; WILKINSON, C. M. Facial Soft Tissue Thickness Database for Craniofacial Reconstruction in Korean Adults. J Forensic Sei, November, v.57, No. 6, 2012

KASAI, K. Soft tissue adaptability to hard tissues in facial profiles. **Am J Orthod Dentofacial Orthop,** Missouri, v.113, p.674-684, 1998.

KOLLMANN, W. J.; BUCHLY, J. Die Persistenz der Rassen und die Reconstructionder Physiognomie Prahistorischer Schadel. Arch Anthropol, v.25, p.329-359, 1898. In:

SAHNI, D.; SANJEEV; SINGH, G.; JIT, L; SINGH, P. Facial soft tissue thickness in northwest Indian adults. **Forensic Sei Int,** Ireland, v.176, p.137-146, 2008.

LEBEDINSKAYA, G. V.; VESELOVSKAYA, E. V. Ultrasonic measurements of the thickness of soft facial tissue among the Bashkirs. **Ann Acad Sei Fenn A,** Helsinki, v. 175, p.91-95, 1986.

MANHEIN, M. H.; LISTI, G. A.; BARSLY, R. E.; MUSSELMAN, R.; BARROW, N. E.; UBELAKER, D. H. In vivo facial tissue depth measurements for children and adults. **J Forensic Sei,** Massachusetts, v.45, p.48-60, 2000.

MIYASAKA, S.; YOSHINO, M.; IMAIZUMI, K.; SETA, S. The computer-aided facial reconstruction system. **Forensic Sei Int,** Ireland, v.74, p. 155-165,1995.

NELSON, L. A.; MICHAEL, S. D. The application of volume deformation to 3-D facial reconstruction: a comparison with previous techniques. **Forensic Sei Int,** Ireland, v.94, p. 167-181, 1998.

PARRA, F.C.; AMADO, R.C.; LAMBERTUCCI, J.R.; ROCHA, J.; ANTUNES, C.M.; PENA, S.D.J. Colour and genomic ancestry in Brasilians. Proc Natl Acad Sei, USA, V.100, n° 1, p. 177-182, 2003.

PANENKOVÁ, P.; BENUS, R.; MASNICOVÁ, S.; OBERTOVÁ, Z.; GRUNT, J. Facial soft tissue thicknesses of the mid-face for Slovak population. **Forensic Sei Int,** Ireland, v.220, p.293.e1-293.e6, 2012.

PERLAZA, N. A. Facial soft tissue thickness of Colombian adults. **Forensic Sei Int,** Ireland, v. 229, p.160.e1-160.e9, 2013.

PHILLIPS, V. M.; SMUTS, N. A. Facial reconstruction: utilization of computerised tomography to measure facial tissue thickness in a mixed racial. **Forensic Sei Int,** Ireland, v.83, p.51-59, 1996.

PLUYM, J. V.; SHAN, W. W.; TAHER, Z.; BEAULIEU, C.; PLEWES, C.; PETERSON, A. E.; BEATTIE, O. B.; BAMFORTH, J. S. Use of magnetic resonance imaging to measure facial soft tissue depth. **Cleft Palate Craniofac J,** Pennsylvania, v.44, p.52-57, 2007.

RHINE, J. S.; CAMPBELL, H. R. Thickness of facial tissues in American blacks. **J Forensic Sei,** Massachusetts, v.25, p.847-858,1980.

SAHNI, D.; SANJEEV; SINGH, G.; JIT, I.; SINGH, P. Facial soft tissue thickness in northwest Indian adults. **Forensic Sei Int,** Ireland, v.176, p.137-146, 2008.

SIMPSON, E.; HENNENBERG, M. Variation in soft tissue thickness on the human face and their relation to craniometric dimensions. **Am J Phys Anthropol,** v.118, p. 121-133, 2002.

SIPAHIOGLU, S.; ULUBAY, H.; DIREN, H. B. Midline facial soft tissue thickness database of Turkish population: MRI study. **Forensic Sei Int,** Ireland, v.219, p.282.e1- 282.e8, 2012.

SMITH, S. L.; BUSCHANG, P. H. Midsagittal facial tissue thicknesses of children and adolescent from Montreal growth study. **J Forensic Sei,** Massachusetts, v.46, p.1294-1302, 2001.

SMITH, S. L.; THROCKMORTON, G. S. A newtechnique for three-dimensional ultrasound scanning of facial tissues. **J Forensic Sei,** Massachusetts, v.49, p.1-7, 2004.

STEPHAN, C. N. Beyond the sphere of the english facial approximation literature: ramifications of german papers on western method concepts. **J Forensic Sei,** Massachusetts, v.51, p. 736-739, 2006.

STARBUCK, J. M.; WARD, R. E. The affect of tissue depth variation on craniofacial reconstructions. **Forensic Sei Int,** Ireland, v.172, p.130-136, 2007.

SUTTON, P. R. N. Bizygomatic diameter: the thickness of the soft tissues over the zygions. **Am J Phys Anthropol,** New Jersey, v.30, p.303-310, 1969.

SUZUKI, K. On the thickness of the soft tissue parts of the Japanese face. **J Anthropol Soe Nippon,** v.60, p.7-11, 1948.

TEDESCHI-OLIVEIRA, S. V.; MELANI, R. F. H.; ALMEIDA, N. H.; PAIVA, L. A. Facial soft tissue thickness of Brazilian adults. **Forensic Sei Int,** Ireland, v.193, p.127.e1- 127.e7, 2009.

TYRRELL, A. J.; EVISON, M. P.; CHAMBERLAIN, A. T.; GREEN, M. A. Forensic three-dimensional facial reconstruction: historical review and contemporary developments. J **Forensic Sei,** Massachusetts, v.42, p.653-661,1997.
UTSUNO, H.; KAGEYAMA, T.; DEGUCHI, T.; YOSHINO, M.; MIYAZAWA, H.; INOUE, K. Facial soft tissue thickness in Japanese female children. **Forensic Sei Int,** Ireland, v.152, p. 101-107, 2005.

UTSUNO, H.; KAGEYAMA, T; UCHIDA, K.; YOSHINO, M.; OOHIGASHI, S.; MIYAZAWA, H.; INOUE, K. Pilot study of facial soft tissue thickness differences among three skeletal classes in Japanese females. **Forensic Sei Int,** Ireland, v.195, p.165.e1- 165.e5, 2010.

VANEZIS, A.; VANEZIS, M.; COMBE, G. M. C.; NIBLETT, T. Facial reconstruction using 3-D Computer graphics. **Forensic Sei Int,** Ireland, v.108, p.87-95, 2000.

YOSHINO, M.; MATSUDA, H.; KUBOTA, S.; IMAIZUMI, K.; MIYASAKA, S.; SETA, S. Computer-assisted skull Identification system using video superimposition. **Forensic Sei Int,** Ireland, v.90, p.231-244,1997.

WELCKER, H. Schiller's Scha"del und Todenmaske, nebst Mittheolungen u"ber Scla del Todenmaske Kants Fr., Vieweg und Sohn, Braunschweig, 1883. In: SAHNI, D.; SANJEEV; SINGH, G.; JIT, I.; SINGH, P. Facial soft tissue thickness in northwest Indian adults. **Forensic Sei Int,** Ireland, v.176, p.137-146, 2008.

WILKINSON, C. M. In vivo facial tissue depth measurements for white British children. **J Forensic Sei,** Massachusetts, v.47, p.459-465, 2002.

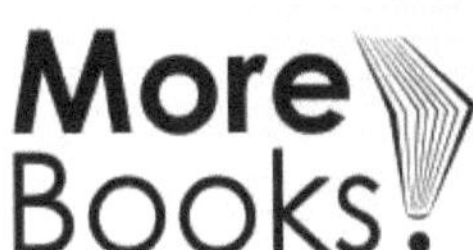

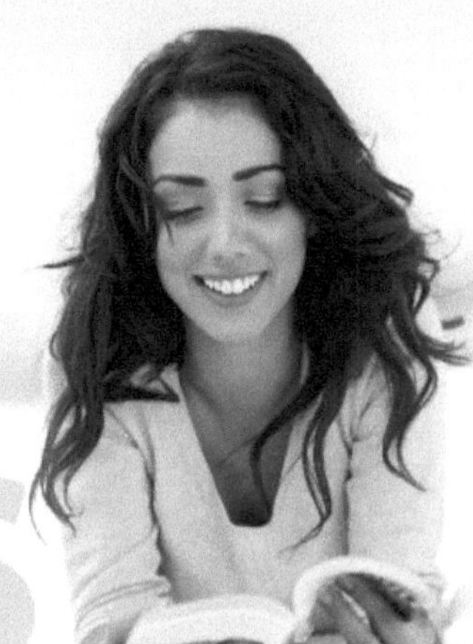

yes
I want morebooks!

Buy your books fast and straightforward online - at one of world's fastest growing online book stores! Environmentally sound due to Print-on-Demand technologies.

Buy your books online at
www.morebooks.shop

Kaufen Sie Ihre Bücher schnell und unkompliziert online – auf einer der am schnellsten wachsenden Buchhandelsplattformen weltweit! Dank Print-On-Demand umwelt- und ressourcenschonend produziert.

Bücher schneller online kaufen
www.morebooks.shop

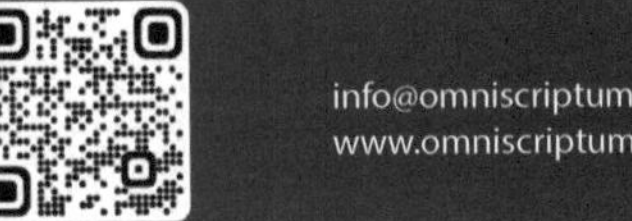

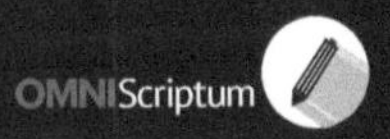

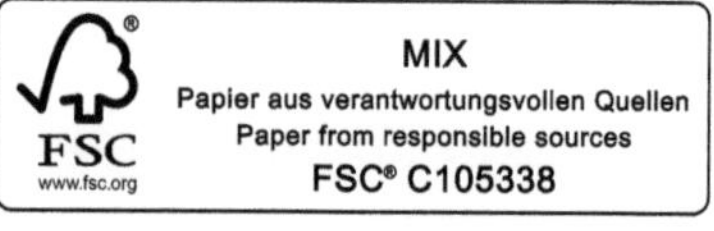

Printed by Books on Demand GmbH, Norderstedt / Germany